GRACIE'S NUTTY  ALLERGY

DAWN PERRIER

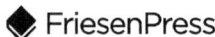

FriesenPress

Suite 300 - 990 Fort St
Victoria, BC, V8V 3K2
Canada

www.friesenpress.com

The content and information within this book is in no way medical or parenting advice and therefore should not be considered as medical or parenting advice. Caregivers must consider what information related to allergies they communicate to children as some of the examples within this book may not be age appropriate some children based on their developmental level or understanding of related topics. Parents and caregivers are encouraged to use their own discretion when explaining concepts within this book to their children.

ISBN
978-1-5255-1032-8 (Paperback)
978-1-5255-1033-5 (eBook)

1. HEALTH & FITNESS, ALLERGIES

Distributed to the trade by The Ingram Book Company

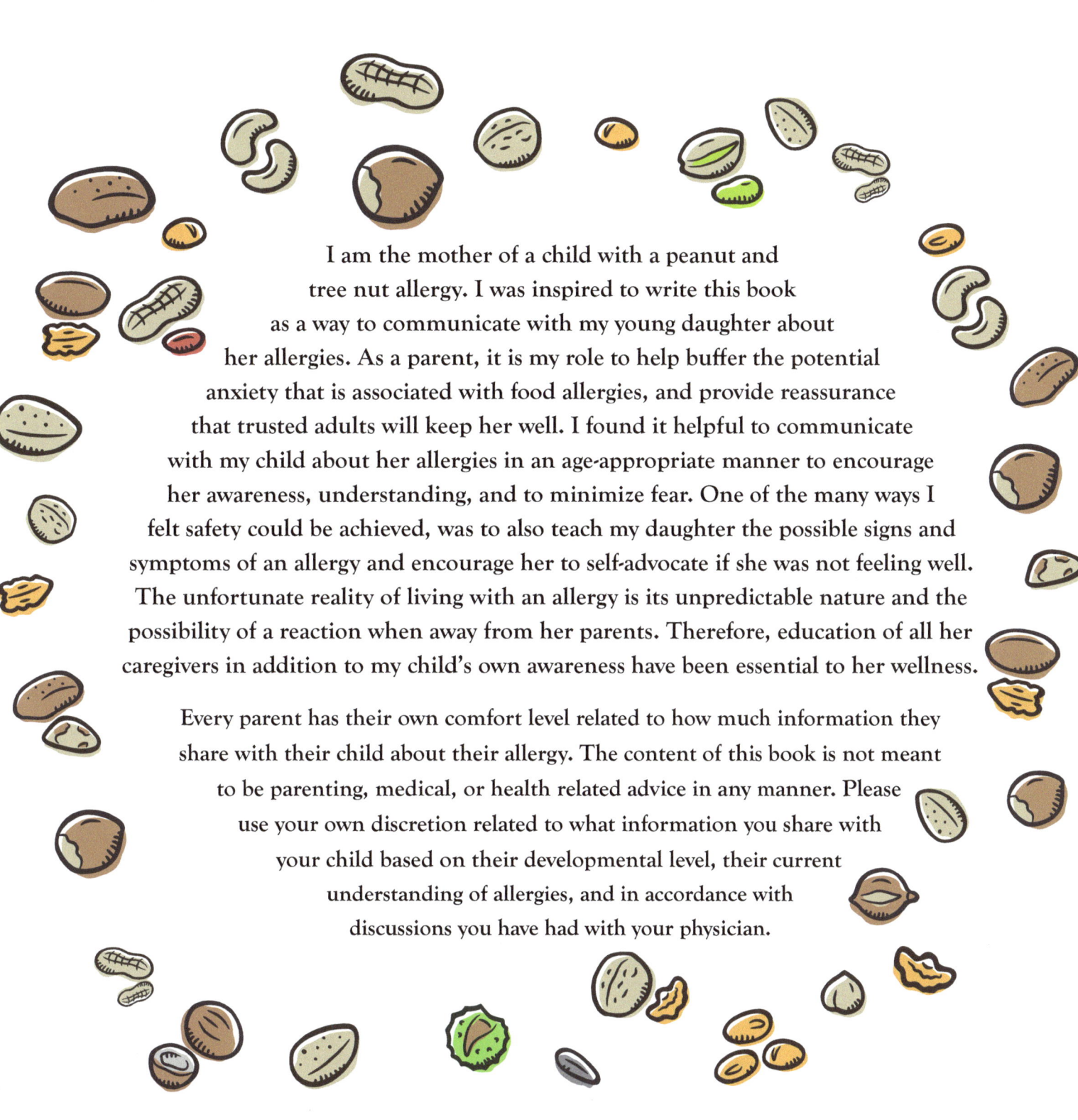

I am the mother of a child with a peanut and tree nut allergy. I was inspired to write this book as a way to communicate with my young daughter about her allergies. As a parent, it is my role to help buffer the potential anxiety that is associated with food allergies, and provide reassurance that trusted adults will keep her well. I found it helpful to communicate with my child about her allergies in an age-appropriate manner to encourage her awareness, understanding, and to minimize fear. One of the many ways I felt safety could be achieved, was to also teach my daughter the possible signs and symptoms of an allergy and encourage her to self-advocate if she was not feeling well. The unfortunate reality of living with an allergy is its unpredictable nature and the possibility of a reaction when away from her parents. Therefore, education of all her caregivers in addition to my child's own awareness have been essential to her wellness.

Every parent has their own comfort level related to how much information they share with their child about their allergy. The content of this book is not meant to be parenting, medical, or health related advice in any manner. Please use your own discretion related to what information you share with your child based on their developmental level, their current understanding of allergies, and in accordance with discussions you have had with your physician.

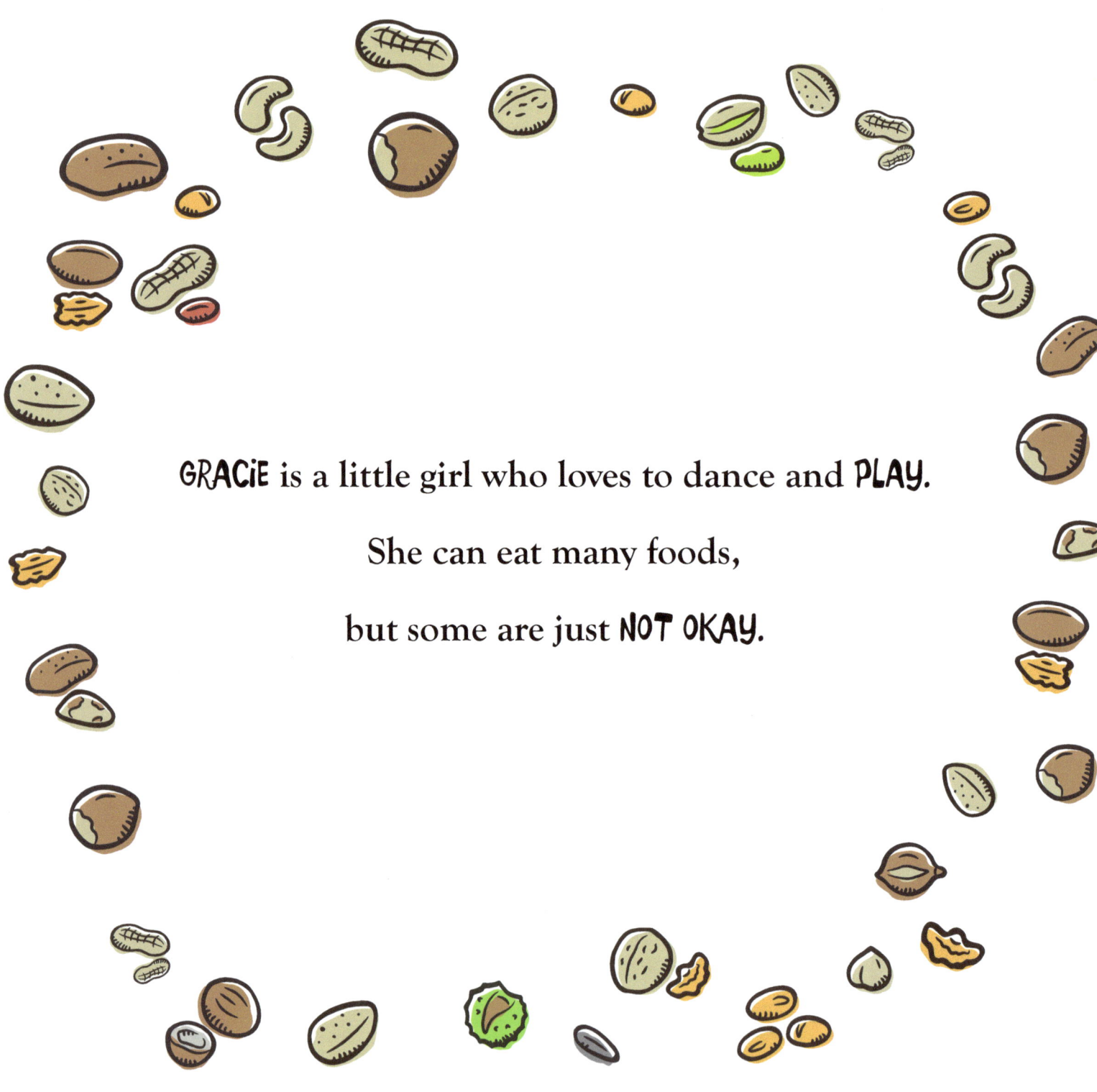

GRACIE is a little girl who loves to dance and PLAY.

She can eat many foods,

but some are just NOT OKAY.

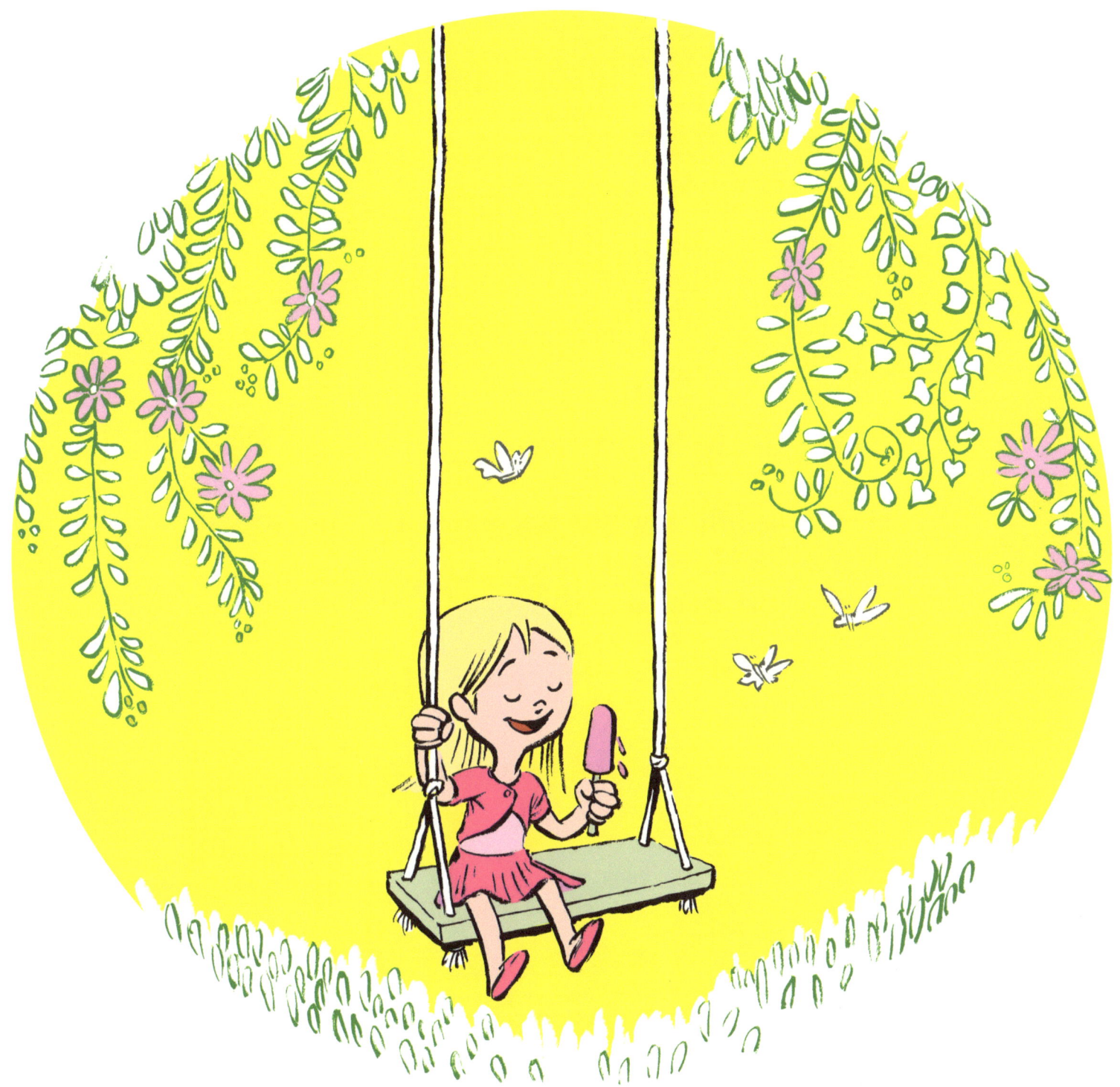

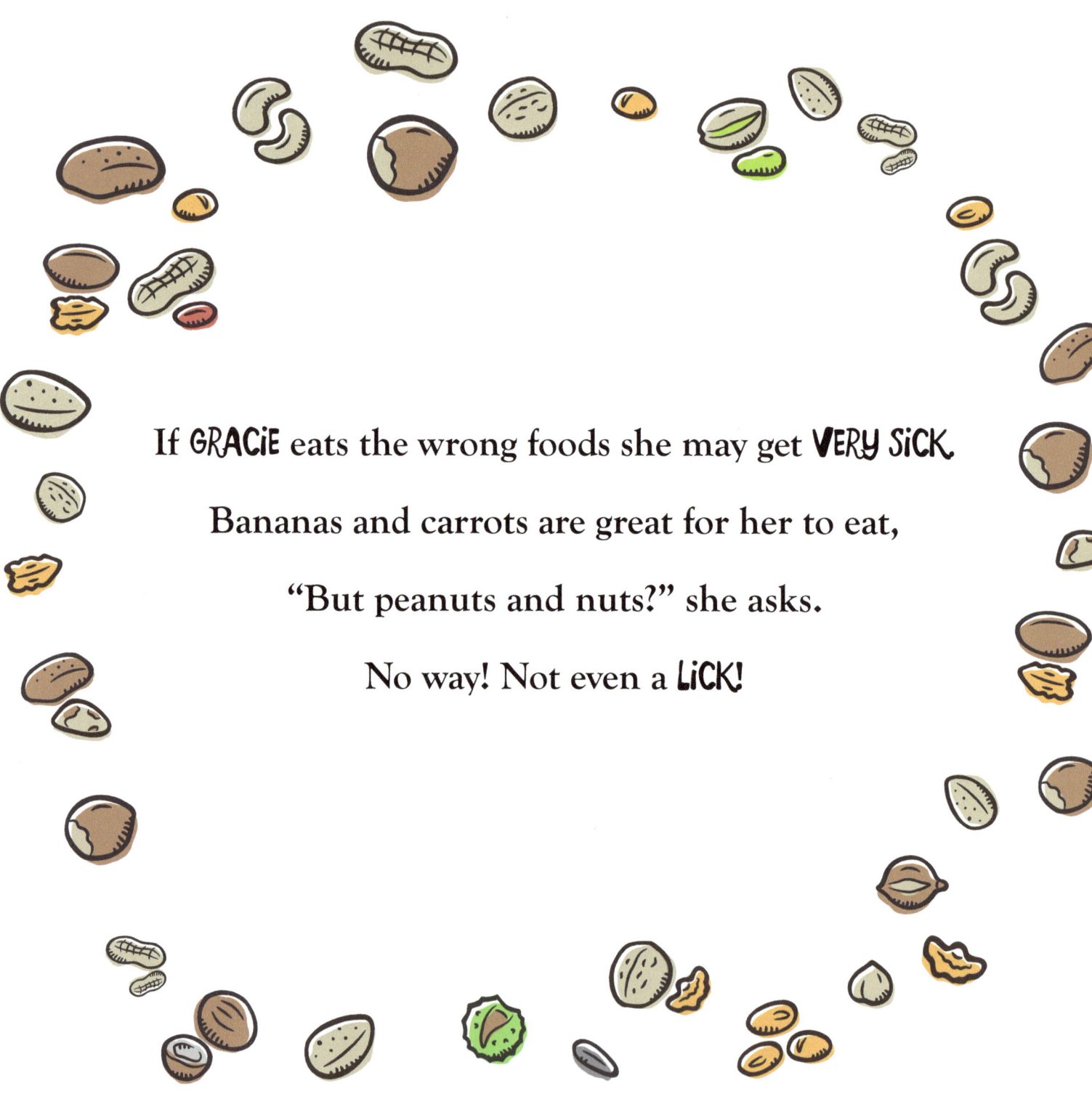

If GRACiE eats the wrong foods she may get VERY SiCK.

Bananas and carrots are great for her to eat,

"But peanuts and nuts?" she asks.

No way! Not even a LiCK!

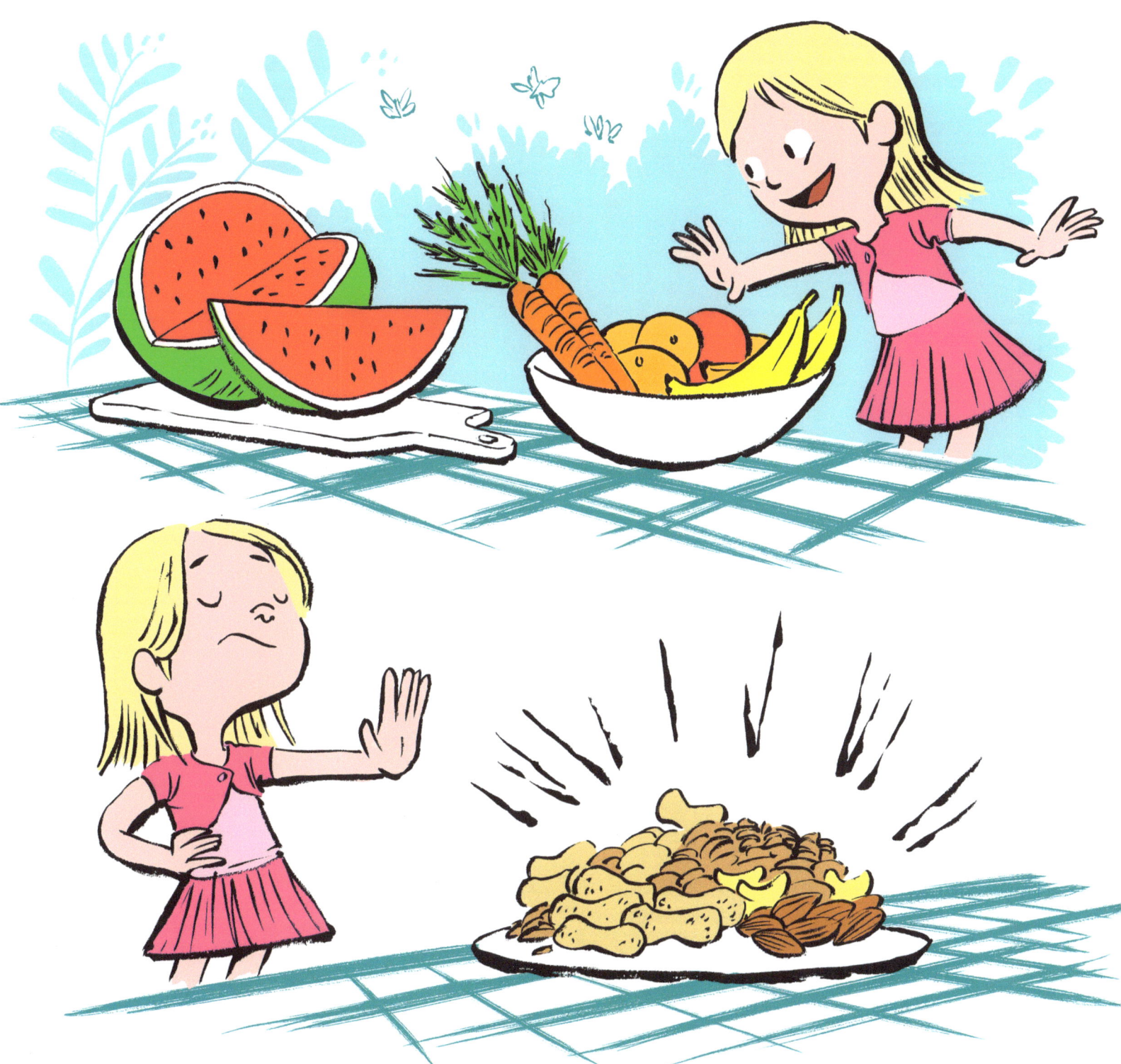

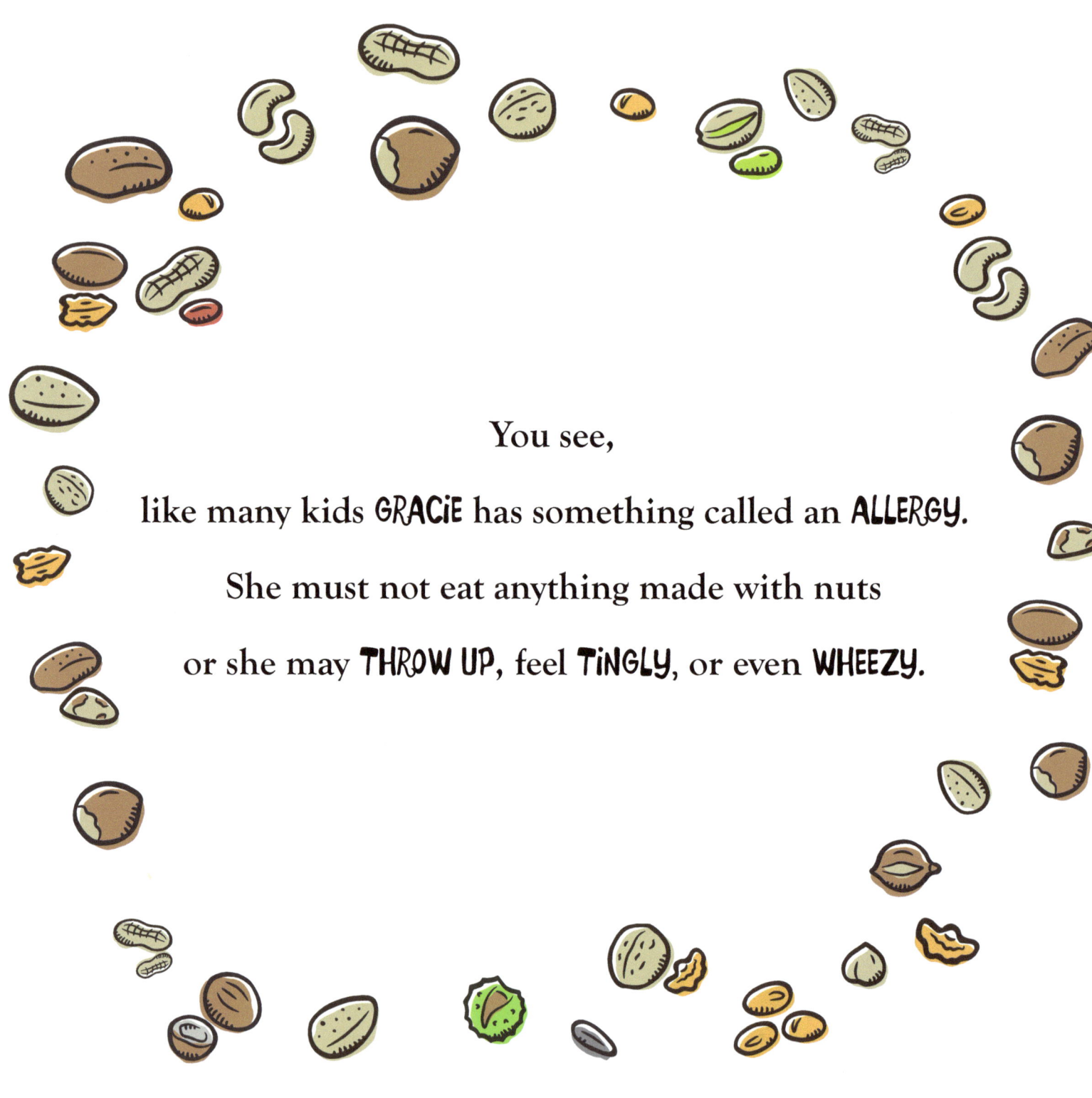

You see,

like many kids GRACiE has something called an ALLERGY.

She must not eat anything made with nuts

or she may THROW UP, feel TiNGLY, or even WHEEZY.

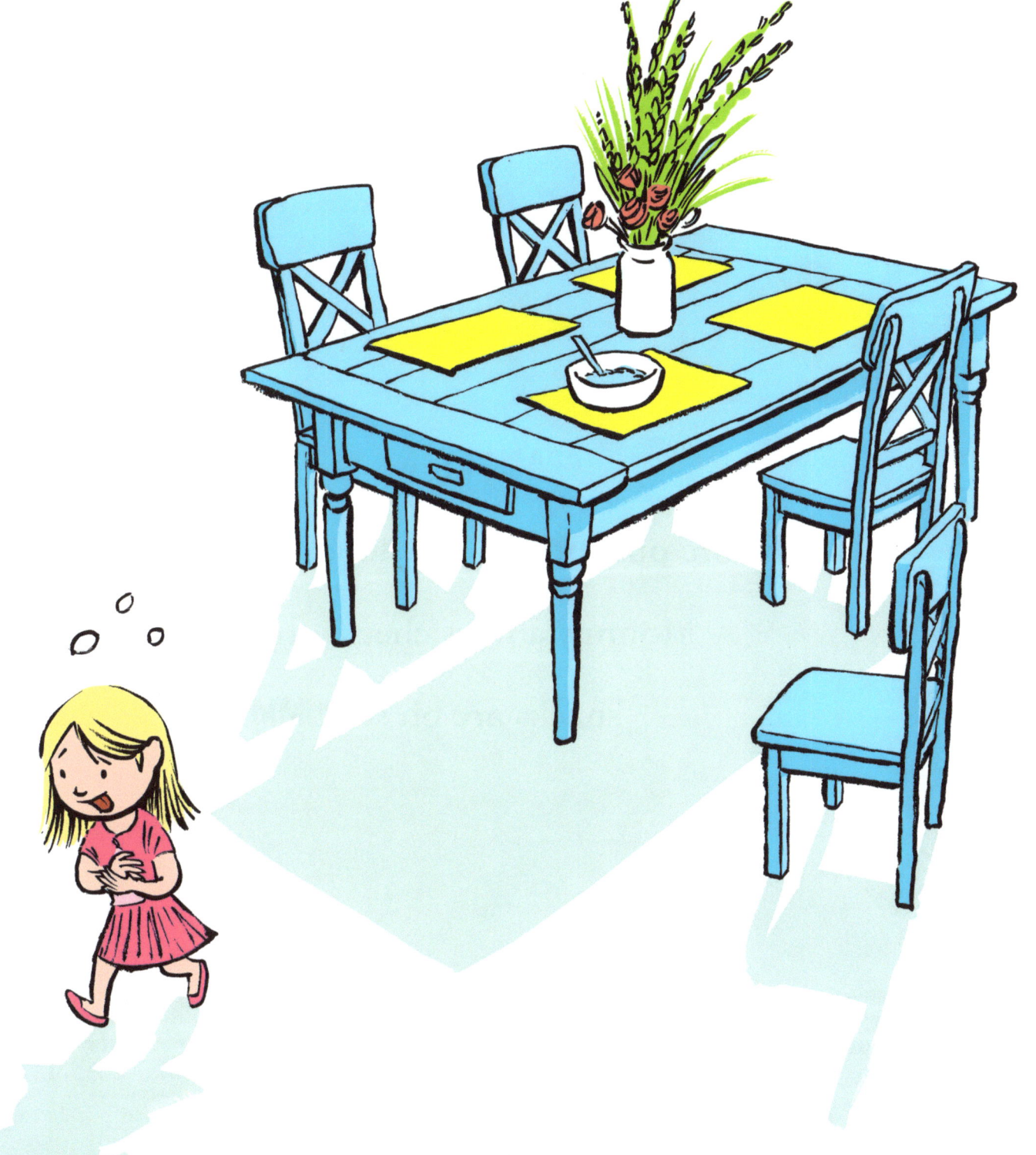

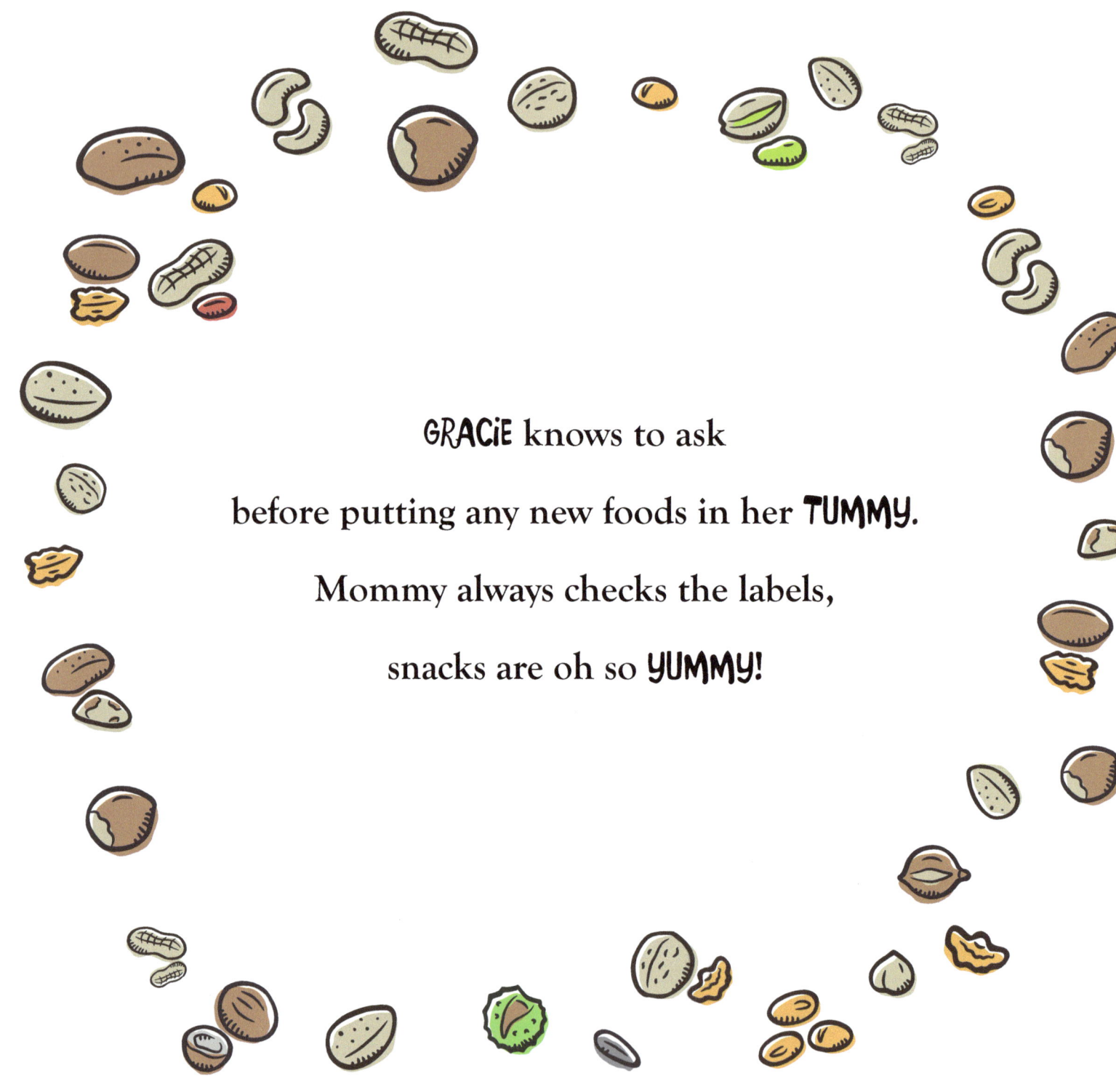

GRACiE knows to ask

before putting any new foods in her TUMMY.

Mommy always checks the labels,

snacks are oh so YUMMY!

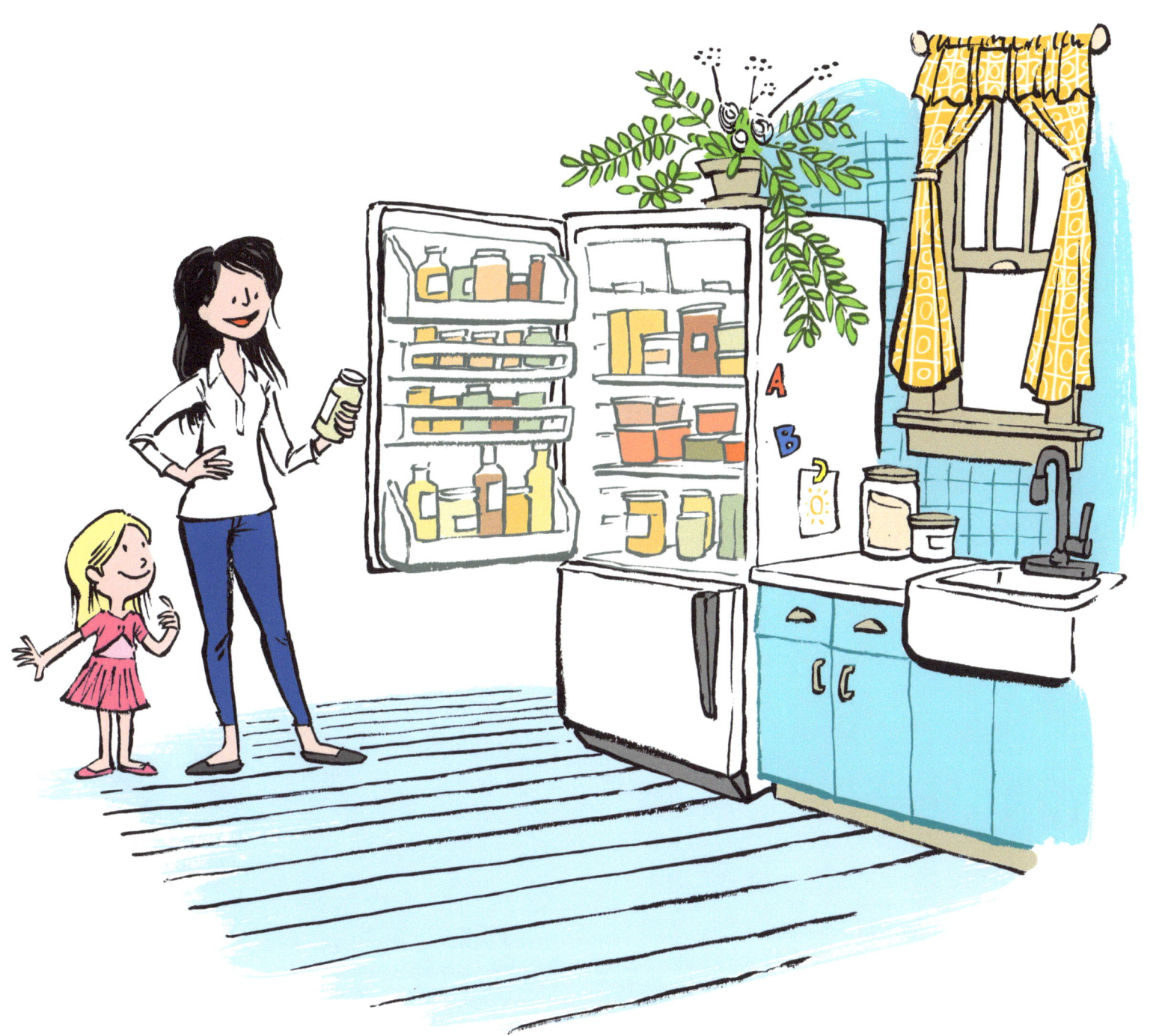

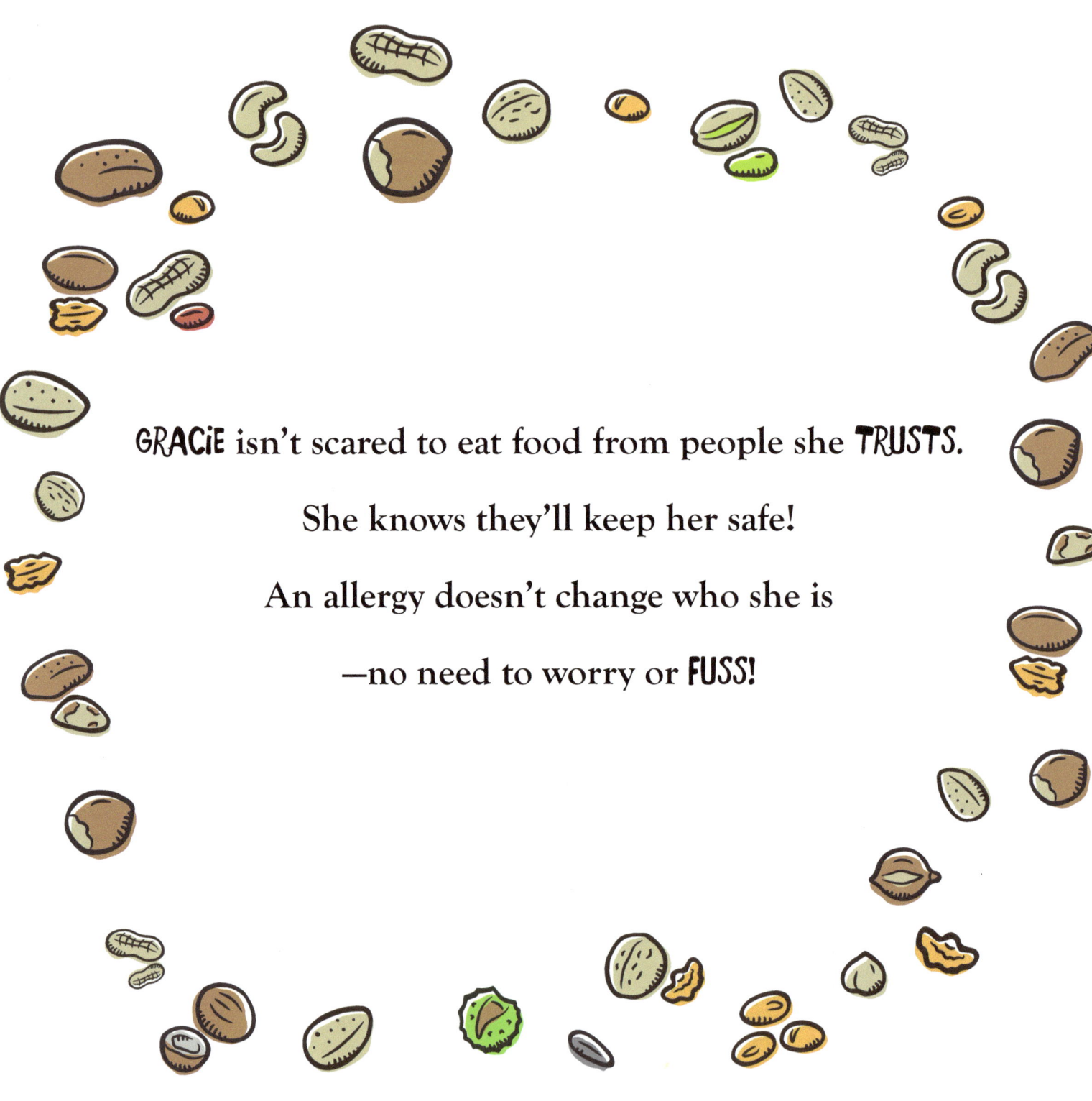

GRACiE isn't scared to eat food from people she TRUSTS.

She knows they'll keep her safe!

An allergy doesn't change who she is

—no need to worry or FUSS!

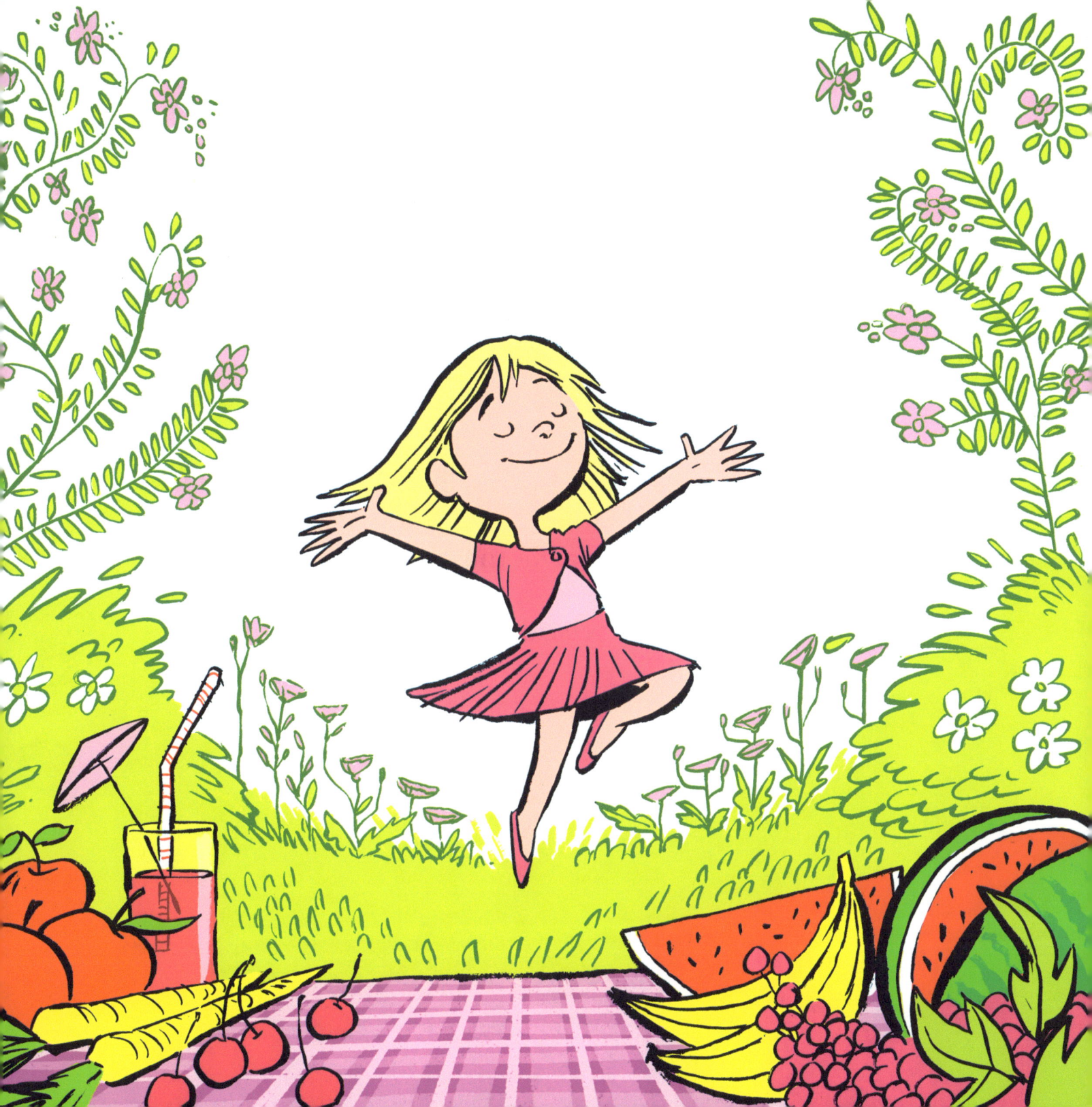

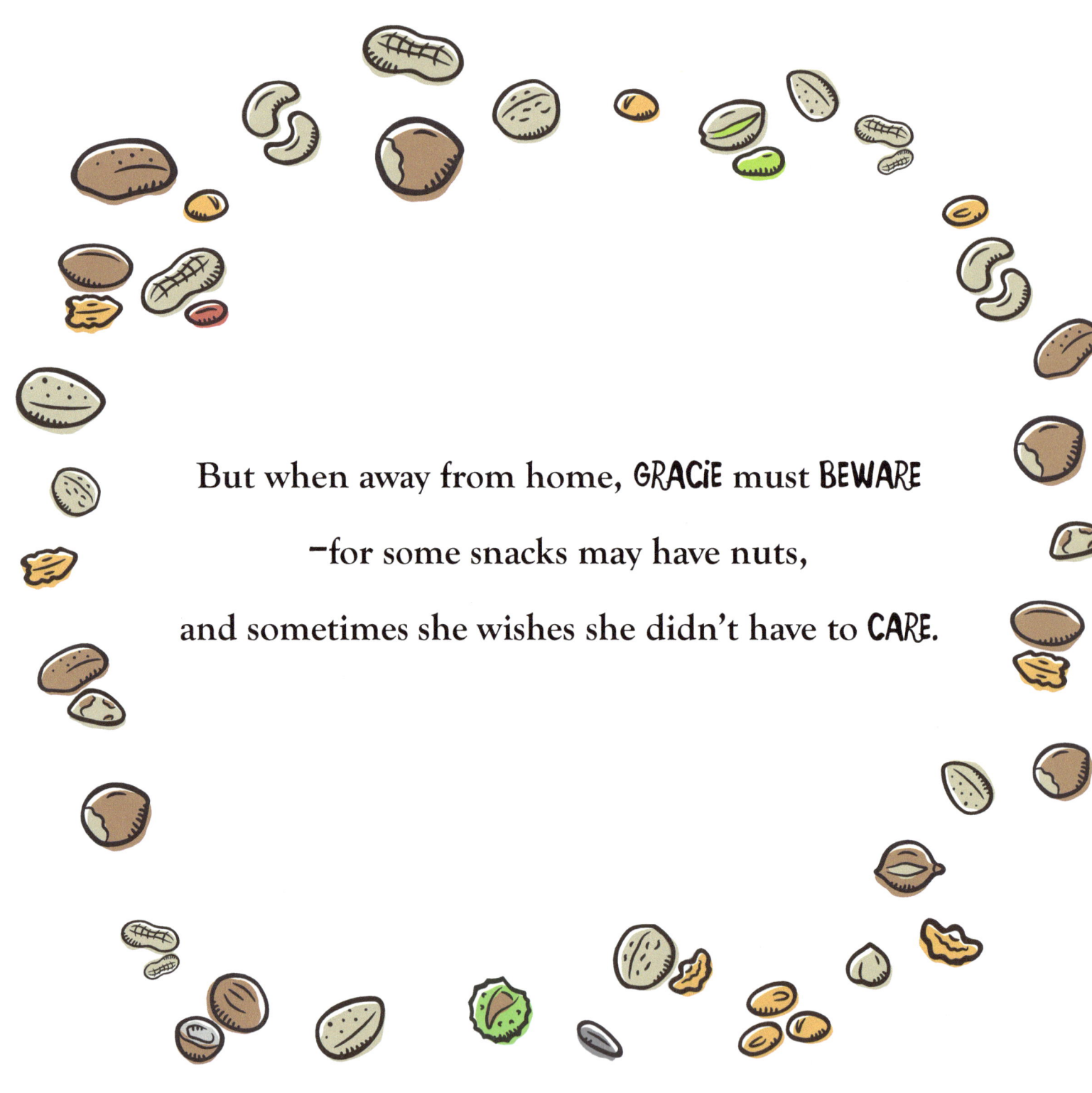

But when away from home, GRACiE must BEWARE

—for some snacks may have nuts,

and sometimes she wishes she didn't have to CARE.

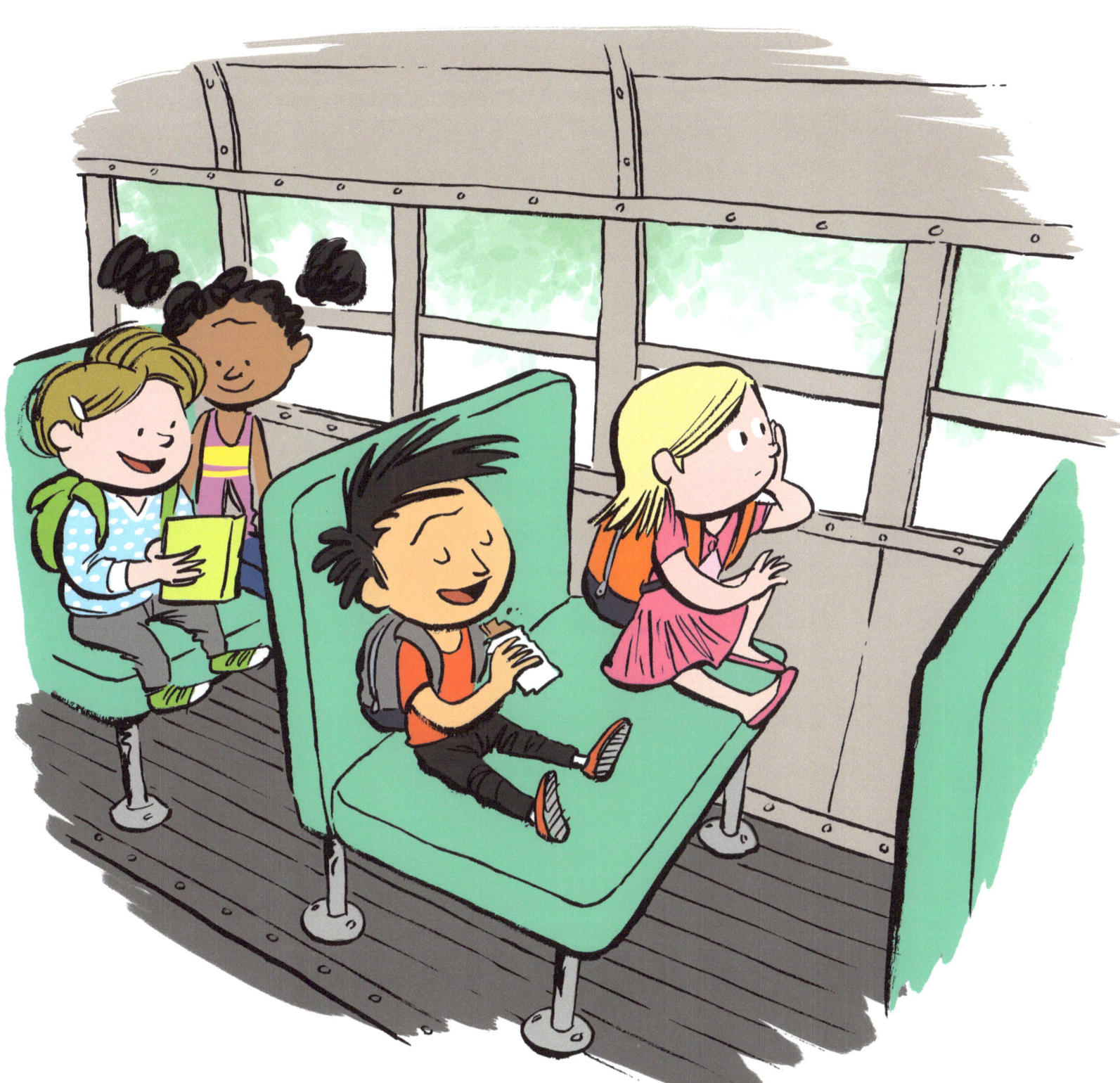

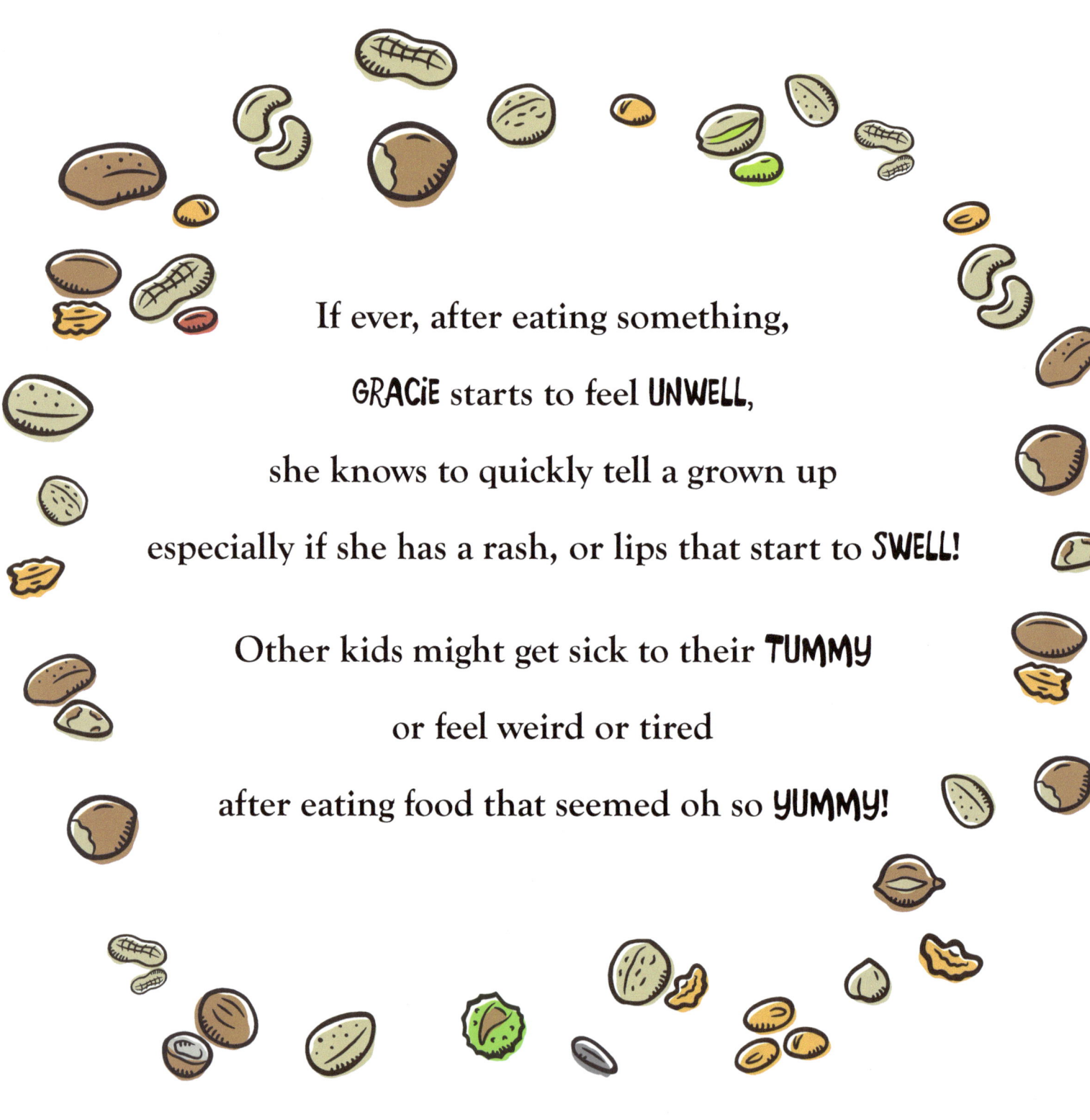

If ever, after eating something,

GRACiE starts to feel UNWELL,

she knows to quickly tell a grown up

especially if she has a rash, or lips that start to SWELL!

Other kids might get sick to their TUMMY

or feel weird or tired

after eating food that seemed oh so YUMMY!

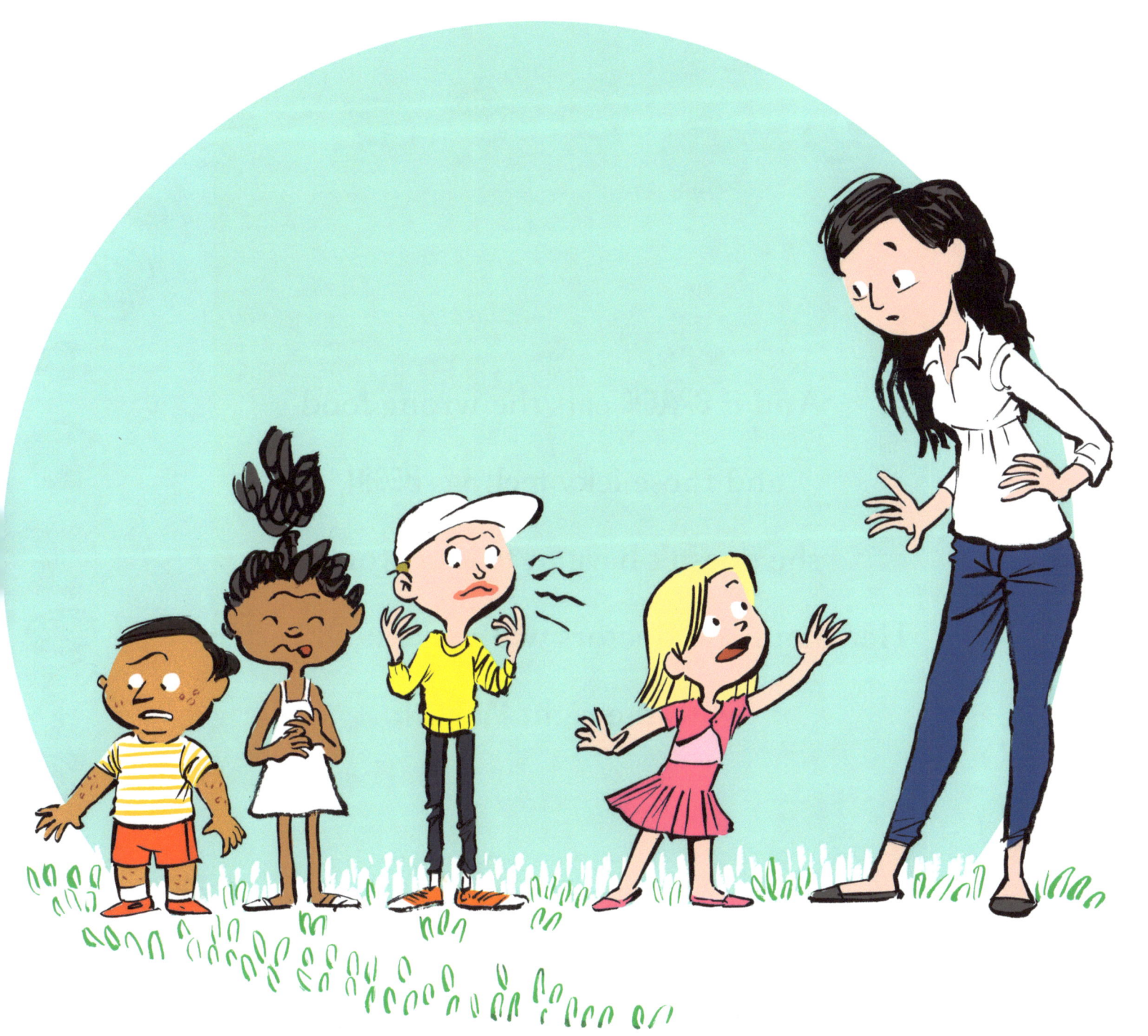

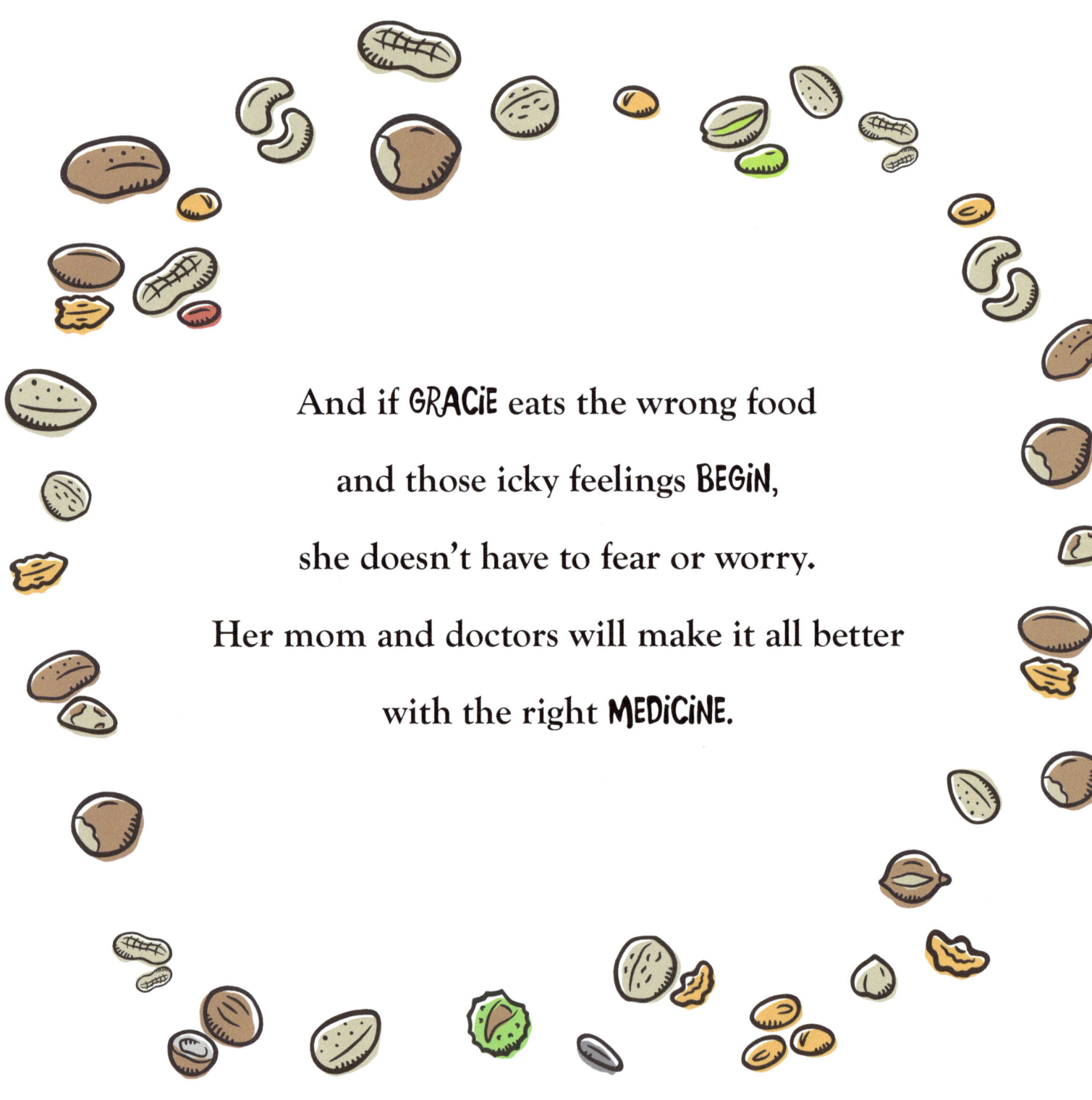

And if GRACiE eats the wrong food

and those icky feelings BEGiN,

she doesn't have to fear or worry.

Her mom and doctors will make it all better

with the right MEDiCiNE.

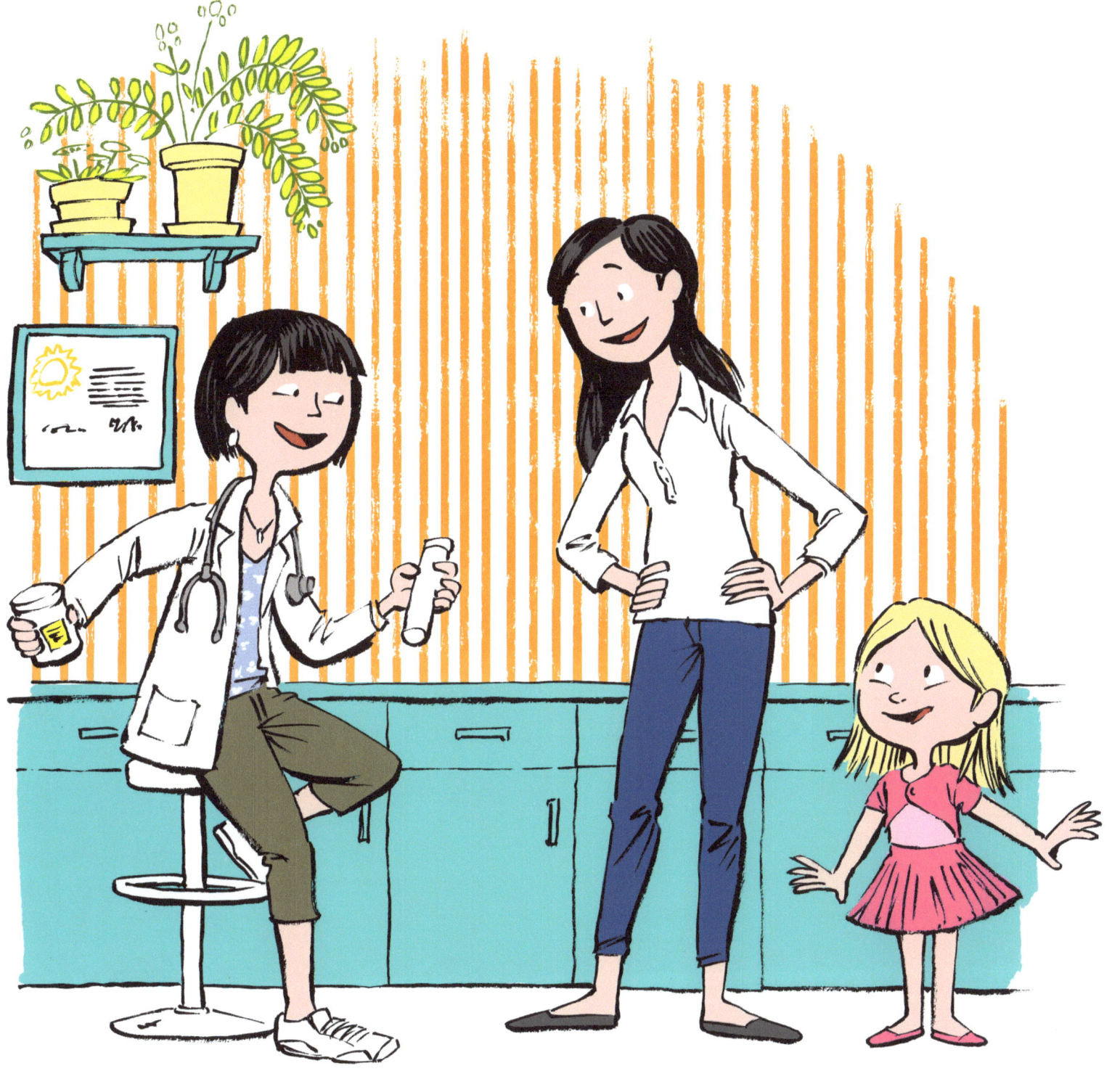

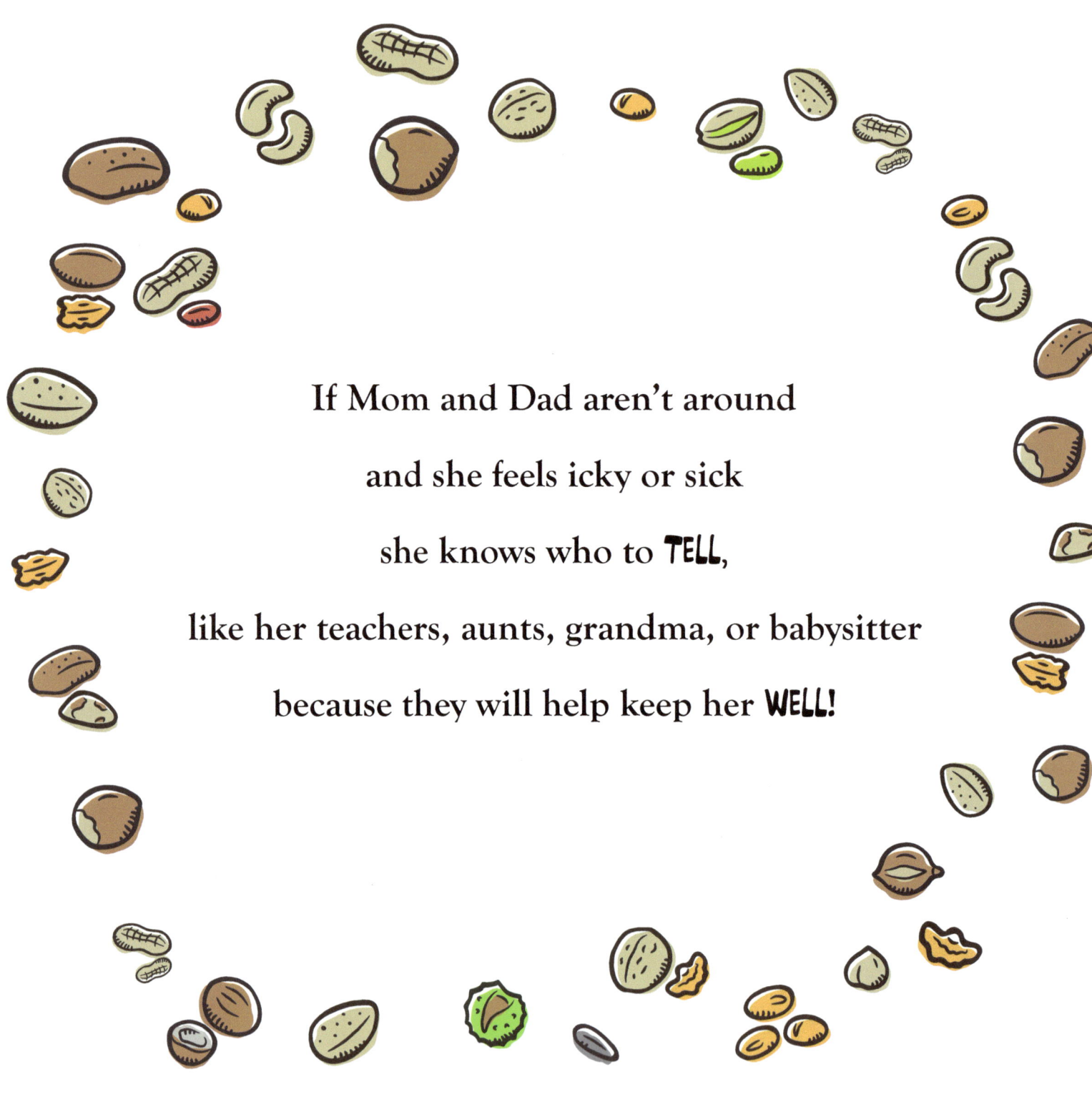

If Mom and Dad aren't around

and she feels icky or sick

she knows who to **TELL**,

like her teachers, aunts, grandma, or babysitter

because they will help keep her **WELL!**

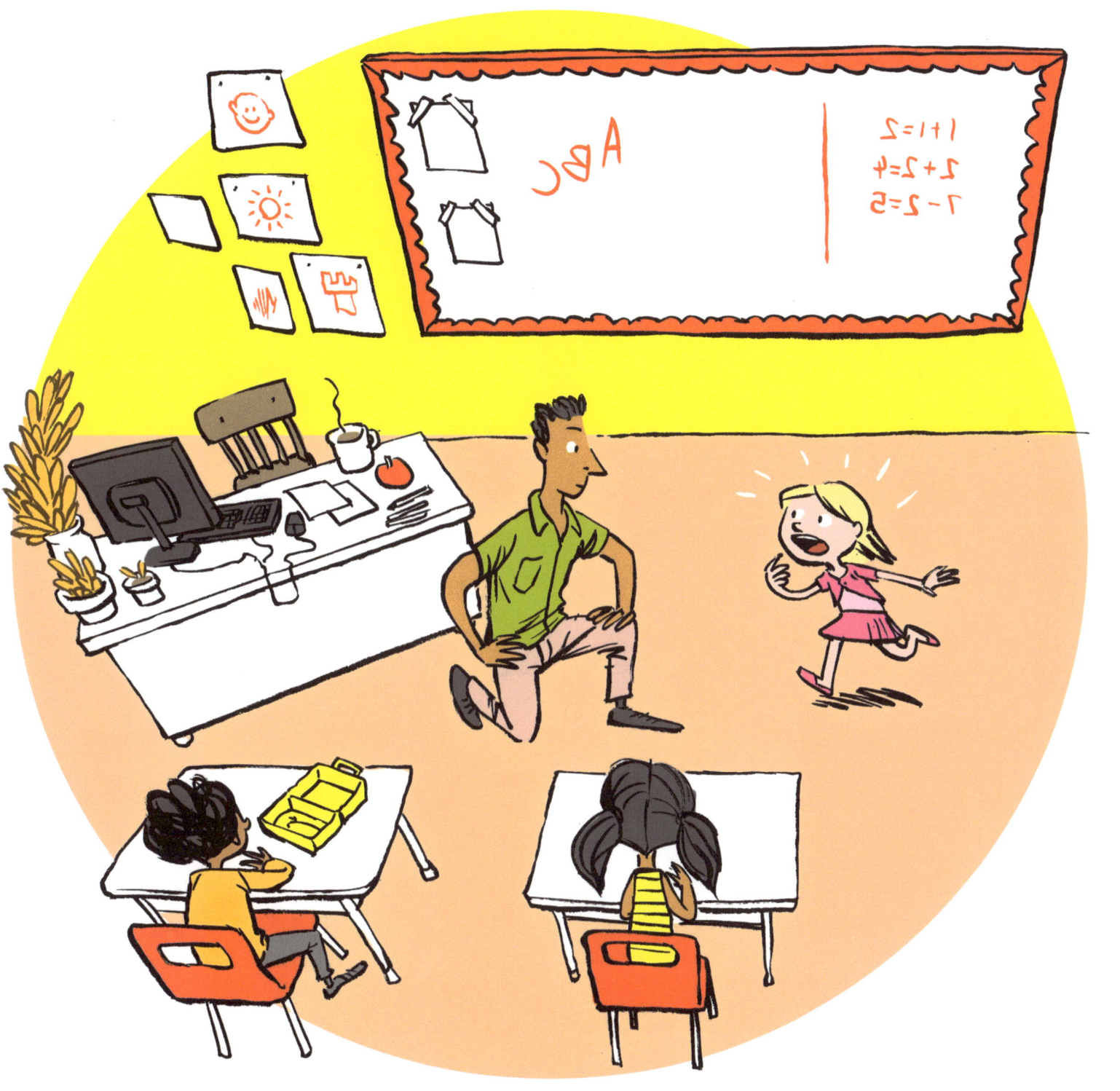

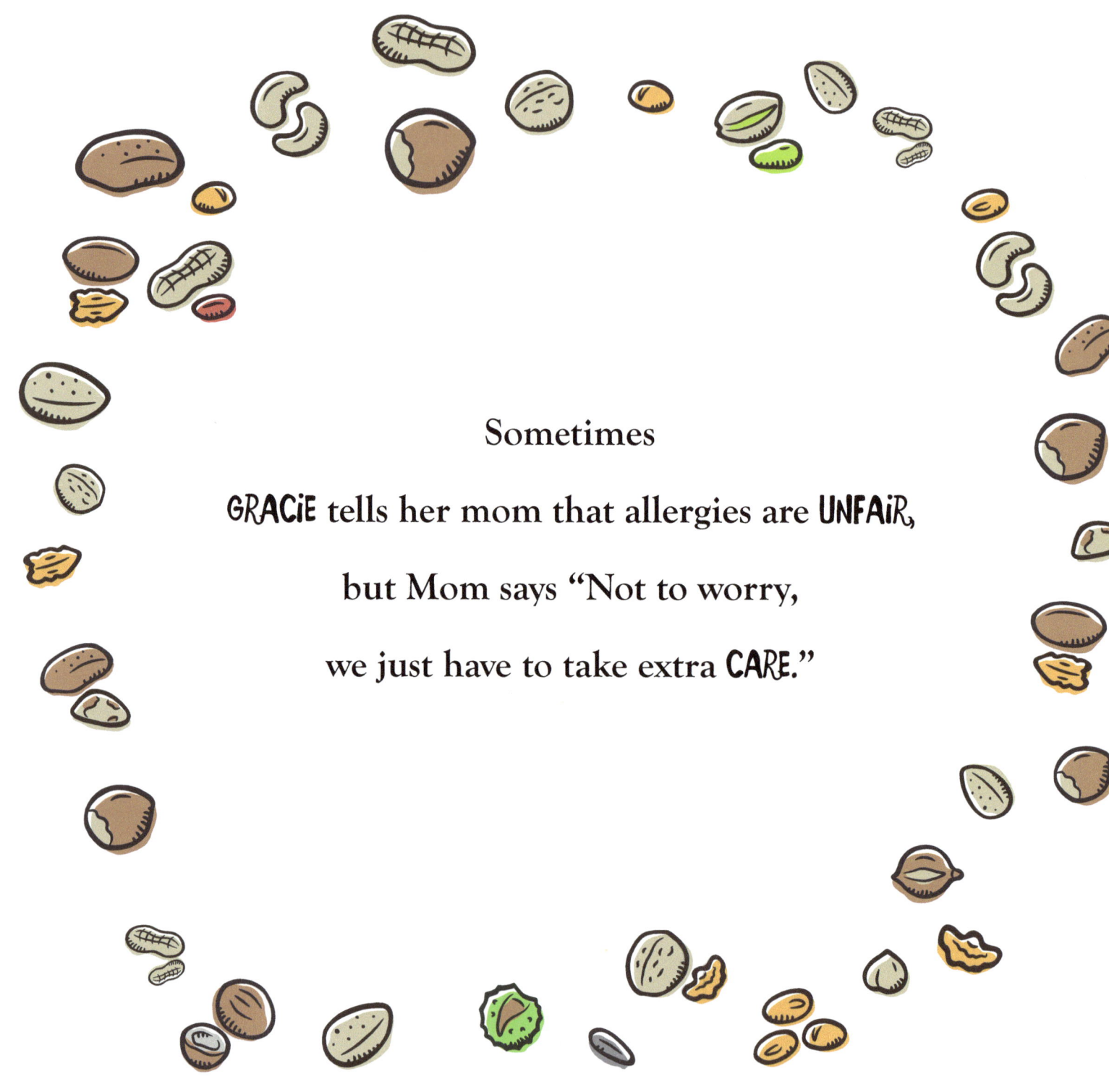

Sometimes

GRACiE tells her mom that allergies are UNFAiR,

but Mom says "Not to worry,

we just have to take extra CARE."

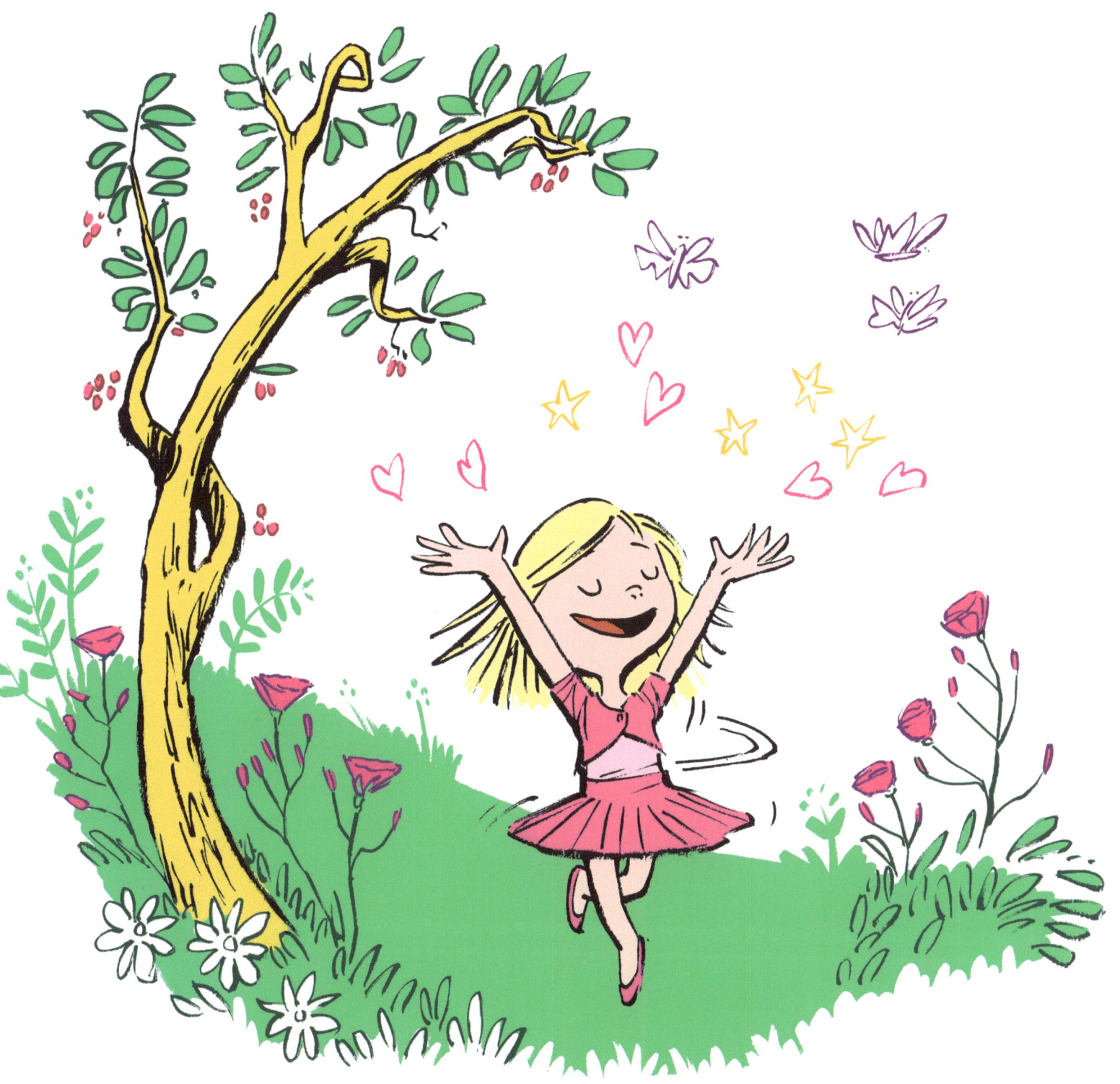

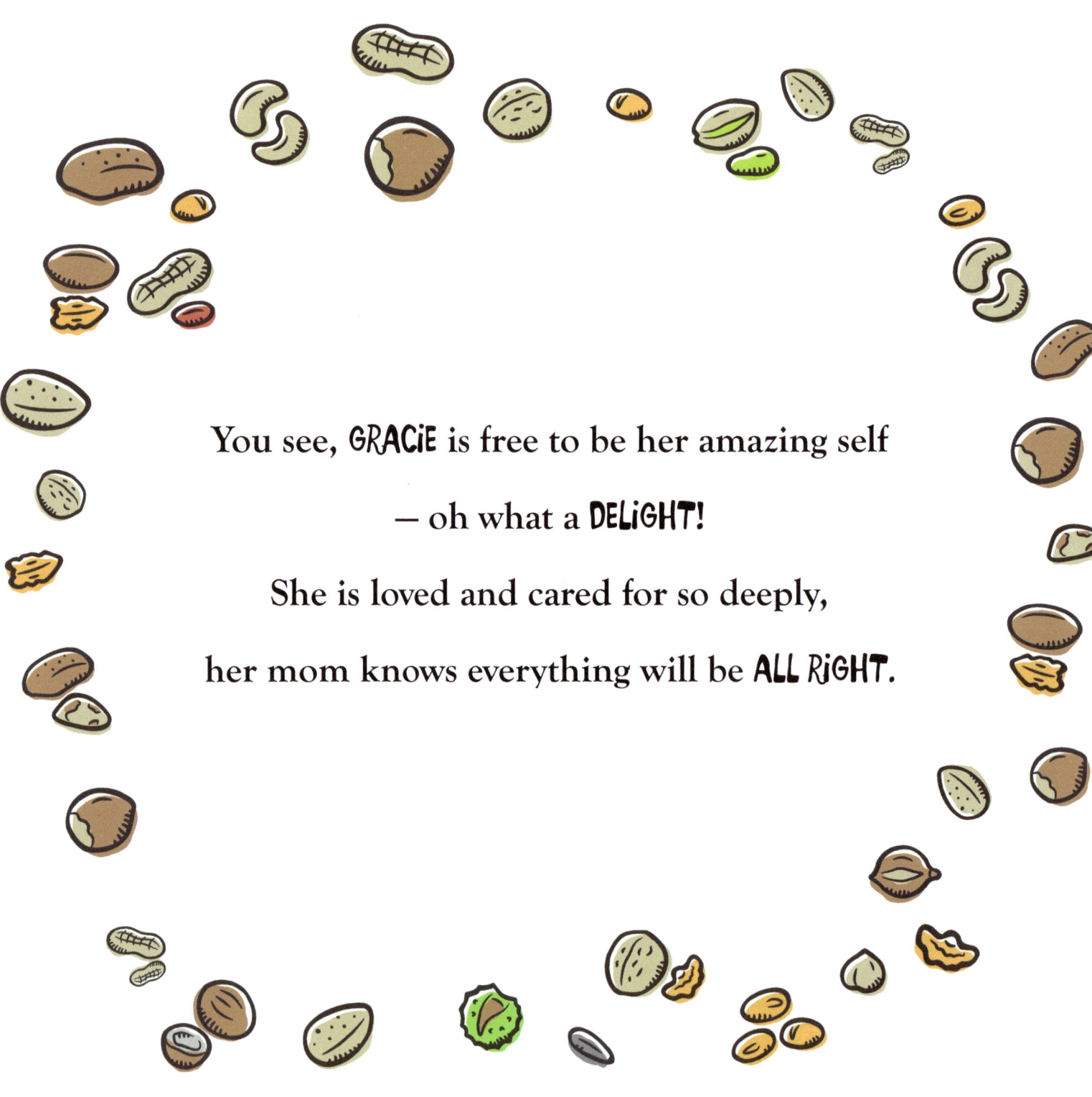

You see, **GRACiE** is free to be her amazing self

— oh what a **DELiGHT!**

She is loved and cared for so deeply,

her mom knows everything will be **ALL RiGHT.**

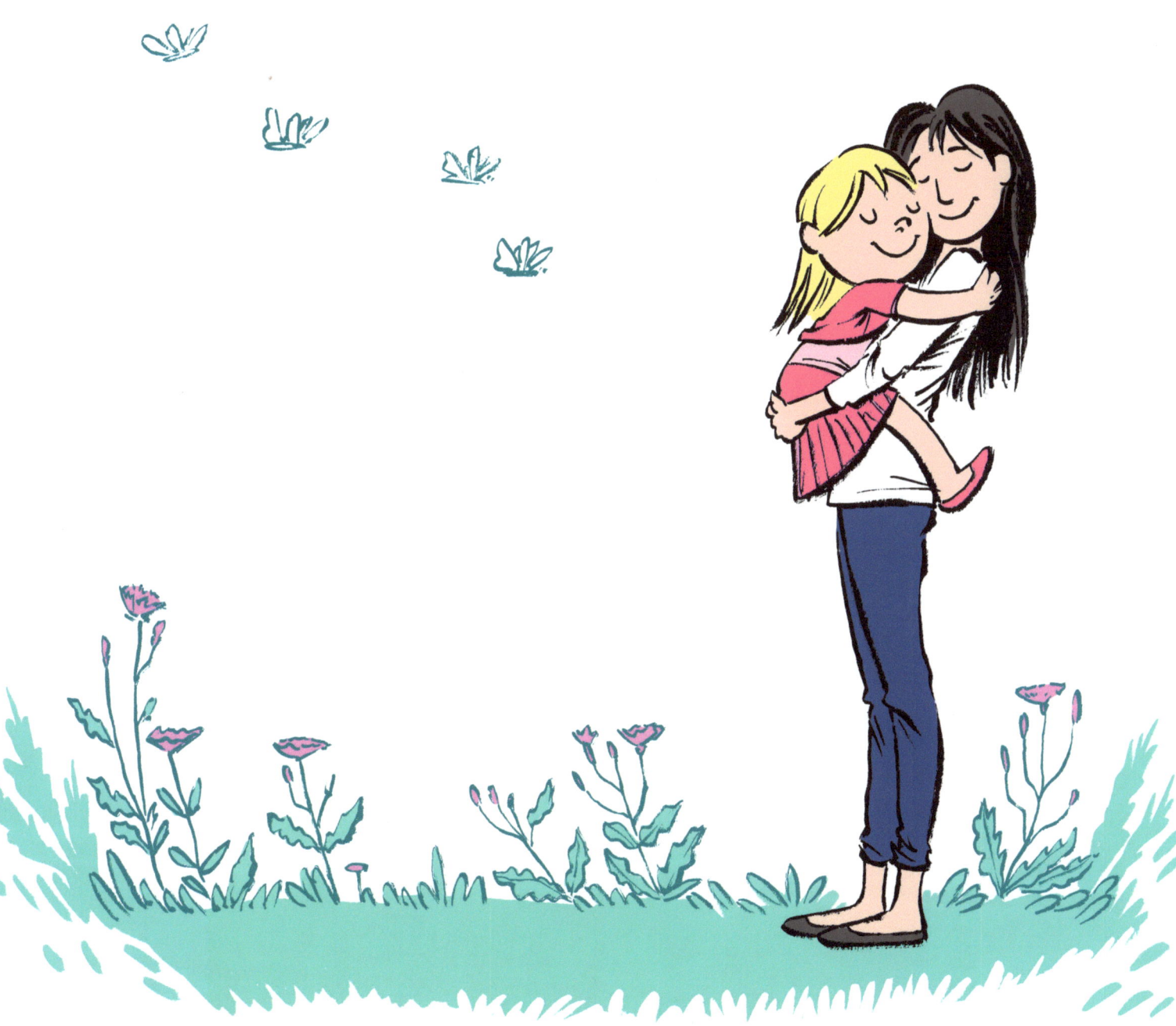

www.ingramcontent.com/pod-product-compliance
Lightning Source LLC
Chambersburg PA
CBHW040309010626
45792CB00025B/1697